DEFEATING IRRITABLE BOWEL SYNDROME (IBS) WITH EXPERT GUIDANCE

Ultimate Solution Handbook For Patients, Guardians Or Family To Understand, Manage, Treat, Prevent, Reverse Symptoms And Live Well

[1]

DR. POTTER WHITLEY

websites, organizations, or other names. The author has no connection to, endorsement from, or recommendation for these organizations. The author's approval or validation is not implied by the inclusion of these references.

Any direct, indirect, incidental, special, or consequential damages resulting from using or not being able to use the material in this book are not covered by the author's liability policy. For medical advice and counsel particular to their circumstances, readers are advised to check with experienced healthcare specialists.

The content, materials, and information in this book are subject to change at any time without prior notice, at the author's discretion. The text may contain errors or omissions for which the author is not responsible.

By reading this book, you understand and accept the conditions of this disclaimer.

THE REASON BEHIND THIS BOOK

An excellent book that tackles the complicated and frequently difficult terrain of irritable bowel syndrome is "Defeating Irritable Bowel Syndrome With Expert Guidance" (IBS). The first section of this book provides readers with a thorough introduction to IBS, highlighting the importance of professional help for managing the condition effectively. It establishes the foundation for a thorough exploration of the nuances of IBS by explicitly defining the goal and parameters of this work.

One important aspect of the study is the examination of IBS, which includes diagnosis, categorization, and common symptoms that might appear in different ways. The significant influence that IBS has on day-to-day living becomes clear to readers, emphasizing the necessity of managing the condition with a comprehensive strategy. The underlying causes and triggers of IBS are painstakingly uncovered in this book, ranging from genetics and biology to psychology and nutrition. It provides readers with a thorough grasp of the complex nature of this disease by accomplishing this.

In particular, the section on diagnosing IBS is quite informative, offering both consumers and medical professionals a road map. This book walks readers through the critical processes involved in correctly diagnosing and treating IBS, from reviewing medical history and symptoms to ordering specific testing and imaging techniques.

The focus this book places on the function of professionals in IBS management makes it stand out. It promotes a team-based approach to therapy by highlighting the knowledge of psychologists, dietitians, and gastroenterologists. This strategy goes beyond the recommended lifestyle changes for IBS, talking about the value of consistent exercise, ways to manage stress, and how good sleep hygiene affects IBS symptoms.

With a thorough examination of the low-FODMAP diet, customized nutrition plans, and the complex connection between gut health and dietary choices, dietary options for managing irritable bowel syndrome (IBS) take center stage. In addition to offering prescription and over-the-counter options, this book also delves into developing therapies and current research on drugs and therapies.

This book gains a holistic quality from the incorporation of supplementary and alternative methods such as herbal supplements, mind-body techniques, and probiotics. It recognizes the range of choices accessible to people looking to reduce their symptoms of IBS.

This thorough book covers important topics such as mental well-being and coping mechanisms. It talks about how IBS affects people emotionally, stresses the value of peer relationships and support networks, and provides helpful tips for developing resilience and keeping an optimistic outlook.

To give persons suffering from IBS hope and encouragement, this book ends with a forward-looking view of future trends and advancements in IBS research.

Essentially, "Defeating Irritable Bowel Syndrome With Expert Guidance" is a source of wisdom and encouragement, giving readers the means to confidently and resolutely traverse the challenging terrain of IBS.

TABLE OF CONTENT

CHAPTER ONE

INTRODUCTION
An Overview Of IBS, Or Irritable Bowel Syndrome:

Irritable Bowel Syndrome, or IBS for short, is a gastrointestinal condition that affects a large percentage of people worldwide. Many symptoms, such as bloating, diarrhea, constipation, and stomach pain, are characteristic. IBS is a chronic illness that severely lowers a person's quality of life and frequently causes emotional and everyday activity disturbances.

IBS is difficult to diagnose and treat because its precise origin is yet unknown. IBS symptoms are thought to develop and worsen in response to a variety of factors, including stress, food, and changes in the gut microbiota. Healthcare professionals and patients with IBS must have a thorough understanding of this syndrome to appropriately manage and alleviate its symptoms.

The numerous IBS subtypes, its diagnostic standards, and the potential psychological and physical consequences for sufferers will all be covered in this section of the book. It seeks to provide readers with a thorough grasp of the syndrome, establishing the foundation for the knowledgeable advice that will be presented in the ensuing chapters.

Expert Advice's Importance For IBS Management

More than a general awareness of IBS is necessary to navigate its complexity. To manage IBS efficiently and enhance the quality of life for people who are impacted, expert guidance is essential. Specialists in gastroenterology can provide individualized treatment regimens, dietary guidance, and psychological support to address the complex nature of irritable bowel syndrome.

The book will stress in this section how crucial it is for anyone suffering from IBS to get professional advice. To give a thorough and individualized treatment plan, it will examine the advantages of a multidisciplinary approach comprising nutritionists, gastroenterologists, and mental health specialists. Being knowledgeable about IBS management entails keeping up with the most recent findings, identifying personal triggers, and utilizing evidence-based treatments to reduce symptoms and improve general health.

The Book's Objective And Scope:

The principal aim of this book is to act as a source of information and assistance for people with IBS. The book attempts to provide readers with the knowledge and skills necessary to take charge of their symptoms and enhance their general quality of life. The book covers more ground than just an outline of IBS; it also explores how to manage and lessen the effects of IBS through lifestyle changes, practical tactics, and the most recent medical developments.

A plethora of knowledge about dietary therapies, stress reduction methods, and IBS-related drugs will be available to readers. Along with offering insights on coping strategies and building resilience, the book will also cover the emotional side of having a chronic illness. It aims to be a complete resource that people, caregivers, and medical professionals may refer to whenever they need help overcoming irritable bowel syndrome.

CHAPTER TWO

KNOWLEDGE OF IRRITABLE BOWEL SYNDROME
The Meaning And Categorization Of IBS:

A group of symptoms affecting the large intestine are the hallmark of the chronic gastrointestinal illness known as irritable bowel syndrome, or IBS. IBS is a common ailment, but because it's so elusive and variable, it can be difficult to diagnose accurately. Clinically, recurring stomach pain or discomfort is used to diagnose IBS in conjunction with changes in bowel habits, such as diarrhea, constipation, or both.

IBS is divided into four subtypes by the Rome Criteria, widely used diagnostic criteria: mixed-type (IBS-M), unsubtyped (IBS-U), IBS with constipation (IBS-C), and IBS with diarrhea (IBS-D). Clinicians can customize treatment techniques for each subtype by using the prevalent bowel pattern as a distinguishing factor.

Recognizing the multifaceted causes of IBS, which include genetic, environmental, and psychological aspects, is essential to understanding the condition. The complex interaction of these components makes diagnosis and treatment more difficult and adds to the variability of IBS presentations. Changes in the two-way connection between the central nervous system and the gastrointestinal tract are critical to the pathophysiology of IBS, which is further highlighted by our growing understanding of the gut-brain axis. Understanding the complex network of factors influencing the onset and evolution of IBS is just as important as understanding its range of clinical presentations.

Typical Signs And Their Changes:

IBS presents with a wide range of symptoms, all of which exacerbate the difficulty in diagnosing the condition. One of the main characteristics is abdominal pain or discomfort, which is frequently eased by feces. Past this point, the range of symptoms varies amongst the subtypes. Frequent loose or watery stools are indicative of IBS-D, whereas infrequent hard stools are indicative of IBS-C.

The symptoms of mixed-type IBS-M are dynamic and change over time, including aspects of diarrhea and constipation. The clinical complexity of IBS is further increased by symptoms like bloating, urgency, and a feeling of incomplete evacuation.

The differences in symptomatology not only make diagnosis more difficult but also highlight the necessity for a customized management strategy. To enable targeted therapies based on the prevailing bowel pattern, effective intervention necessitates a detailed understanding of the unique symptoms that each experience. IBS symptoms are erratic and can be triggered by food, stress, and other factors.

As such, a treatment plan that is flexible and dynamic is required. Clinicians are better able to hone their diagnostic skills and provide more targeted therapies as research reveals the complex pathways behind IBS symptoms.

IBS has a significant impact on afflicted individuals' daily lives in addition to its medical symptoms. Because the symptoms are erratic, social, professional, and recreational activities may be severely disrupted. Because the illness is chronic, people struggle with the ongoing uncertainty of when their symptoms can flare up. This further compounds the condition's negative effects. It is important to recognize the psychological toll that IBS takes, as anxiety and depression frequently coexist with the physical symptoms.

IBS sufferers may have to strike a careful balance between controlling their symptoms and continuing to lead somewhat normal lives. A lower quality of life is caused by the need for frequent restroom stops, dietary limitations, and the psychological toll that comes with having a chronic illness. People may struggle with social connections and work productivity as a result of the stigma and misinformation around IBS. The close relationship between mental health and gut health emphasizes the significance of treating IBS holistically, which includes not only treating the physical symptoms but also the emotional and social factors that have a big influence on day-to-day functioning. The rising complexity of IBS is making it more and more important for healthcare professionals and researchers to develop interventions that address both the physiological and psychosocial aspects of the illness to lessen its far-reaching impacts.

CHAPTER THREE

IBS CAUSES AND TRIGGERS AT THEIR CORE
Genetics and Biological Elements:

It takes a thorough analysis of biological variables and genetic predispositions to comprehend the underlying causes and triggers of irritable bowel syndrome (IBS). A person's genetic composition is frequently the cause of the complex gastrointestinal illness known as IBS. There is a substantial hereditary component to IBS, as evidenced by research showing that those with a family history of the ailment are more likely to develop it themselves.

Abnormalities in the structure and function of the gastrointestinal tract are among the many biological variables that contribute to IBS. The symptoms of IBS are caused by several factors, including irregular motility, increased sensitivity of the intestines, and changes in the gut-brain communication system. These biological anomalies have the potential to cause discomfort, bloating, and irregular bowel movements by causing the intestinal muscles to contract irregularly.

Furthermore, comprehending the basic foundations of IBS requires a comprehension of the complex interactions between the immune and neurological systems. Serotonin is one neurotransmitter that is important in controlling gut function. IBS is frequently linked to altered serotonin levels, which impact sensation and bowel movement.

In conclusion, the development of IBS is facilitated by biological variables and genetic predispositions. Understanding the complexities of the molecular and genetic components offers important new perspectives on possible therapeutic modalities for the management and treatment of IBS.

Factors related to psychology and stress:

There is a complex and reciprocal interaction between psychological factors and Irritable Bowel Syndrome (IBS). It is often known that psychological stress is a cause of IBS symptoms, and people with IBS frequently have an increased sensitivity to stressors. An important factor in this relationship is the brain-gut axis, which is a communication network that connects the gut with the central neurological system.

IBS symptoms can be made worse by stress and emotions, which have a substantial impact on gut health. Prolonged stress can cause visceral hypersensitivity, changes in the gut microbiota, and changes in gut motility, all of which can contribute to the development and aggravation of IBS. Furthermore, a common pathophysiology is indicated by the fact that people with IBS frequently report co-occurring disorders like anxiety and sadness.

The psychosocial component of IBS is also influenced by behavioral and cognitive variables. The severity of symptoms and the overall effect that IBS has on a person's quality of life can be influenced by negative thought patterns, coping strategies, and conditioned responses.

In summary, a knowledge of IBS that takes into account the complex interactions between psychological factors and the condition is essential. It may be possible to manage IBS and enhance the general well-being of those who experience it by addressing psychological issues through therapeutic methods like cognitive-behavioral therapy.

Nutritional Affects:

Dietary factors are found to be important in both the onset and aggravation of Irritable Bowel Syndrome (IBS). Certain food triggers that might cause or exacerbate symptoms are frequently mentioned by IBS sufferers. For efficient management and symptom relief, it is crucial to comprehend these dietary influences.

IBS symptoms have been linked to specific kinds of carbohydrates called fermentable oligosaccharides, disaccharides, monosaccharides, and polyols (FODMAPs). These poorly absorbed carbohydrates may ferment in the digestive tract, producing gas, causing bloating, and changing the habits of the bowels. As such, some IBS sufferers have found that following a low-FODMAP diet helps to reduce their symptoms.

Apart from FODMAPs, dietary variables including fat consumption and food allergies could also be involved in the symptoms of IBS. High-fat meals have the potential to cause changes in bowel habits and abdominal pain by inducing colonic contractions. While not always present in IBS patients, food allergies or intolerances can also contribute to the expression of symptoms.

People with IBS must follow a customized diet plan that is overseen by a medical expert or certified dietitian. The general quality of life and symptom control of individuals with IBS can be greatly improved by identifying particular dietary triggers and putting focused dietary adjustments into practice.

Gut Microbiota's Function:

An important field of research that sheds insight on the complex interaction between the microbial communities living in the gastrointestinal system and the development of IBS symptoms is the involvement of gut microbiota in Irritable Bowel Syndrome (IBS). Comprising trillions of bacteria, the gut microbiota is essential for preserving immune system performance, intestinal homeostasis, and general health.

Individuals with IBS have been shown to have dysbiosis or changes in the makeup and activity of the gut microbiota. Irritable bowel syndrome (IBS) symptoms may arise and persist due to alterations in the microbial community's general balance as well as the prevalence of certain bacterial species. This interaction is further complicated by the bidirectional contact between the gut bacteria and the gut-brain axis.

Research indicates that intestinal motility, visceral hypersensitivity, and immunological responses may be impacted by dysbiosis in IBS, resulting in the typical symptoms of bloating, abdominal discomfort, and irregular bowel movements. Furthermore, the low-grade inflammation frequently seen in some IBS patients may be influenced by the interplay between the immune system and the gut flora.

Probiotics and prebiotics are two examples of therapies whose effects on the gut microbiota are being studied as a potential means of treating IBS symptoms. Beneficial bacteria called probiotics may help restore microbial balance, reduce discomfort, and enhance general gut health.

Conclusively, comprehending the function of gut microbiota in IBS offers significant perspectives on plausible treatment approaches. By highlighting the complex interactions between the host and gut bacteria in gastrointestinal health, tailored therapies that target the gut microbiota offer a viable approach to controlling and treating IBS.

CHAPTER FOUR

IDENTIFICATION OF THE IRRITABLE BOWEL SYNDROME
Medical Background and Symptom Evaluation:

Conducting a thorough medical history and symptom assessment is a critical initial step in the diagnosis of Irritable Bowel Syndrome (IBS). Obtaining an extensive medical history enables medical practitioners to comprehend the patient's general state of health, recognize possible risk factors, and investigate the beginning and development of symptoms. Doctors frequently inquire about a patient's food habits, degree of stress, and any triggers that can make their symptoms worse. It is through this procedure that medical professionals may distinguish IBS from other gastrointestinal problems and develop a more individualized treatment plan.

Since IBS is characterized by a variety of gastrointestinal symptoms, symptom assessment is an important part of the treatment. Bloating, changes in bowel habits (constipation, diarrhea, or a combination of both), and stomach pain or discomfort are frequently reported by patients. Sorting IBS into its subtypes, including IBS-D (predominantly diarrhea), IBS-C (predominantly constipation), or IBS-M (mixed bowel habits), is made easier by having a clear understanding of the precise nature and frequency of these symptoms. Treatment plans are also guided by how these symptoms affect the patient's day-to-day functioning, which aids in determining the severity of the ailment.

Laboratory Testing And Physical Examinations:

A comprehensive physical examination is performed to find any physical indicators of IBS or other gastrointestinal disorders after the medical history and symptom assessment are finished. Palpating the belly to feel for soreness, bloating, or unusual lumps is one method of performing a physical examination.

Furthermore, medical professionals could examine general abdominal muscle tone and look for indications of dietary deficits.

Exclusion of other possible causes of gastrointestinal problems is mostly dependent on laboratory testing. Blood tests can be performed to check for anomalies such as anemia and inflammation. Analyses of stool samples can be used to rule out occult blood, parasites, and diseases. Although inflammatory bowel diseases (IBD), celiac disease, or colorectal cancer are ailments that can resemble symptoms of IBS, these tests are necessary to rule them out to rule out IBS itself. IBS itself usually does not cause substantial changes in laboratory results.

Imaging Procedures And Specialized Tests:

Certain tests and imaging methods could be advised if the diagnosis is still unclear or if the patient has unusual symptoms. These tests can offer further information about how the gastrointestinal system is operating.

Hydrogen breath testing, for instance, is useful in detecting glucose malabsorption, a disorder that may exacerbate the symptoms of irregular bowel movements. A colonoscopy or flexible sigmoidoscopy can be used to view the colon and rule out any structural irregularities or other digestive issues.

Comprehensive images of the digestive system can be obtained by imaging techniques including magnetic resonance imaging (MRI) or abdominal computed tomography (CT) scans.

These tests can help find any inflammatory disorders or anatomical anomalies that may be causing the patient's symptoms. These techniques are not usually the first line of diagnostic instruments, but they become useful when underlying structural abnormalities are suspected or when traditional approaches fail to yield a definitive diagnosis.

To sum up, diagnosing Irritable Bowel Syndrome accurately requires a multimodal strategy that includes a detailed medical history, evaluation of symptoms, physical examination, and a tiered approach to laboratory testing, specialist testing, and imaging procedures.

This thorough assessment enables medical professionals to customize treatment regimens to meet the unique requirements and symptoms of every patient.

CHAPTER FIVE

THE EXPERT'S FUNCTION IN IBS ADMINISTRATION
The Specialization of Gastroenterologists:

To treat Irritable Bowel Syndrome (IBS) completely, gastroenterologists are essential. These individuals bring a plethora of expertise and experience to the table as digestive system specialists in medicine. They have made significant contributions, one of which is the reliable diagnosis of IBS through a methodical assessment of symptoms, medical history, and occasionally diagnostic testing. Because the symptoms of IBS and other gastrointestinal illnesses frequently overlap, accuracy is essential.

In addition to diagnosing, gastroenterologists use their knowledge to customize treatment regimens for each patient. They can suggest taking medicine to treat symptoms including bloating, irregular bowel movements, and stomach pain. Furthermore, they can distinguish between distinct IBS subtypes, which guarantees that specific symptom patterns are addressed in treatment plans.

For example, a patient with IBS who experiences constipation more often than diarrhea might be given different advice than someone with diarrhea-predominant IBS.

Following up with gastroenterologists regularly enables continuous evaluation and necessary modifications to treatment regimens. They advise lifestyle changes and keep an eye out for any issues, in addition to managing medications. Additionally, gastroenterologists are an invaluable resource for patients, providing information about breakthroughs in research and treatment alternatives.

In summary, gastroenterologists' knowledge is fundamental to managing IBS because they can offer patients a tailored, multifaceted treatment plan that targets the illness's underlying causes as well as its symptoms.

Dietitians and Advice Regarding Nutrition:

A key component of the multidisciplinary management strategy for irritable bowel syndrome (IBS) involves dietitians. These professionals offer patients priceless advice on how to recognize and control trigger foods because nutrition has a substantial impact on gastrointestinal function. Dietitians utilize the documented correlation between specific food components, like fermentable carbohydrates (FODMAPs), and the symptoms of irritable bowel syndrome (IBS) to develop individualized meal plans.

Before providing individualized nutritional counsel, a complete evaluation of the patient's eating preferences, symptom patterns, and nutritional requirements is necessary. Dietitians collaborate with patients to pinpoint particular foods that can aggravate symptoms and those that can be consumed to support healthy digestive systems. One well-known strategy that limits the consumption of certain carbs known to elicit symptoms of IBS is the low-FODMAPS diet.

Additionally, dietitians educate and support patients continuously, enabling them to make knowledgeable eating decisions. They assist in overcoming obstacles like meal planning, eating out, and keeping a healthy diet despite dietary limitations. Dietitians keep up with the latest research because it is always changing, which means that their advice is supported by evidence and in line with the most recent knowledge on nutrition and IBS.

In the end, dietitians' work requires more than just following a rigid diet; it also entails helping patients develop a healthy and long-lasting connection with food, which enhances general well-being and digestive health.

Mental Health Support and Psychologists:

Psychologists are essential to the comprehensive treatment of Irritable Bowel Syndrome (IBS) because they understand the complex relationship that exists between the mind and the gut. Support for mental health is essential since emotional and stress-related variables can greatly affect the frequency and intensity of IBS symptoms. In addition to providing ways to control stress, anxiety, and other emotional elements that may increase symptoms, psychologists collaborate with patients to study the psychological components of their condition.

Cognitive-behavioral therapy (CBT), which has shown promise in lowering IBS symptoms and enhancing general quality of life, is one of the main therapies used by psychologists. Patients who experience increased stress and discomfort can better understand and change the negative thought patterns and actions that contribute to them. Psychologists contribute to a more thorough and long-lasting treatment approach by treating the psychological aspects of IBS.

Psychologists are also sympathetic listeners who offer a secure environment for patients to voice worries and frustrations associated with managing a chronic illness. Improving the patient's coping skills and resilience can be greatly aided by this emotional support.

A comprehensive approach to managing IBS is ensured with the participation of psychologists and other healthcare specialists. Patients can better navigate the problems associated with IBS and have an enhanced quality of life when the physical and psychological aspects of the condition are addressed.

Collaborative Therapy Approach:

The best way to manage Irritable Bowel Syndrome (IBS) is to work with a team and combine the knowledge of different medical specialists. A group of experts, including psychologists, nutritionists, gastroenterologists, and other medical professionals, collaborate to treat the various facets of IBS and offer all-encompassing therapy in a collaborative paradigm.

This method acknowledges the complex character of IBS and the multiple influences on its genesis and symptomatology, including nutritional, psychological, and physiological variables. As the principal medical specialists, gastroenterologists oversee the patient's physical well-being, prescribe medication, and use diagnostic tools to coordinate the entire treatment plan.

Dietitians provide their specific expertise in nutrition, modifying dietary regimens to control symptoms and enhance digestive well-being. Their knowledge of trigger foods and how to help patients make dietary adjustments is crucial for the long-term management of symptoms.

When it comes to managing stress, worry, and other emotional issues that might aggravate symptoms, psychologists are essential in treating the psychological component of IBS. Along with improving the patient's general well-being, cognitive-behavioral therapy (CBT) and other treatment modalities help to provide a more comprehensive understanding of the disease.

The healthcare team members' regular coordination and communication make sure that every facet of the patient's condition is taken into account. The treatment plan can be modified in response to the patient's changing needs and reactions thanks to this collaborative approach.

A more tailored and sophisticated approach that targets the distinct mix of variables causing their IBS is beneficial to the patients.

Conclusively, an interdisciplinary approach to managing IBS signifies an emphasis on holistic treatment, acknowledging that the illness transcends its somatic manifestations. Patients receive a comprehensive and customized treatment plan that increases the chance of symptom relief and long-term well-being by utilizing the experience of gastroenterologists, nutritionists, psychologists, and other healthcare specialists.

CHAPTER SIX

LIFESTYLE ADJUSTMENTS FOR IBS
The Value of Consistent Exercise

To control and reduce the symptoms of Irritable Bowel Syndrome (IBS), regular exercise is essential. Physical activity has been associated with a host of health advantages, and it can be particularly beneficial to the general well-being of those with IBS. By enhancing the digestive system's effective operation, exercise helps control bowel motions. Food and waste are more easily passed through the intestines when the gastrointestinal tract's muscles are stimulated.

Additionally, regular exercise helps reduce stress, which is a major cause of the symptoms of IBS. Physical activity is a natural way to decrease stress, and it is well-recognized that stress exacerbates IBS symptoms. Exercise triggers the release of endorphins, a class of neurotransmitters that lower stress and increase emotions of enjoyment. Abdominal pain, bloating, and irregular bowel movements may lessen in frequency and severity for those with IBS who incorporate a regular exercise regimen.

Exercise also helps one maintain a healthy weight, which is crucial for controlling IBS. By keeping a healthy weight, you can lessen the chance of aggravating your IBS symptoms and spare your digestive tract further strain. Frequent exercise also aids in the regulation of hormone balance, particularly those that affect digestion, which may help people with IBS live in a more stable environment.

Aerobic exercises that involve walking, running, or cycling can be very helpful for those with IBS. Engaging in these exercises improves overall gastrointestinal function in addition to cardiovascular health. However, it's crucial to customize exercise regimens to each person's tastes and skills because rigorous workouts might exacerbate symptoms for certain IBS sufferers.

In summary, a key element of lifestyle changes for controlling IBS is consistent exercise. Its beneficial effects on digestion, stress reduction, and weight management all add up to help those who are struggling with this illness live better lives.

Methods of Stress Management

Since stress is known to aggravate the symptoms of Irritable Bowel Syndrome (IBS), managing stress is essential to managing IBS effectively. There exist multiple approaches to reduce stress and, in turn, lessen its effects on digestive health. Mindfulness meditation is among the most popular stress-reduction strategies.

People with IBS may find it easier to break the pattern of stress and symptom worsening by practicing mindfulness meditation, which is focusing on the present moment without passing judgment. It has been demonstrated that frequent mindfulness meditation lowers the psychological and physiological effects of stress, fostering a more at-ease state of being. Programs that focus on reducing stress through mindfulness include techniques including progressive muscle relaxation, guided visualization, and deep breathing exercises.

Cognitive-behavioral therapy (CBT) has also shown promise in the treatment of IBS symptoms brought on by stress. Through cognitive behavioral therapy (CBT), people can recognize and alter harmful thought patterns and behaviors that lead to stress. CBT gives IBS patients useful coping mechanisms to handle life's obstacles and lessens the negative effects of stress on their digestive systems by addressing the cognitive and emotional components of stress.

People with IBS may also benefit from practicing relaxation techniques like yoga or tai chi. These mind-body techniques promote balance and tranquility by combining attentive breathing, physical activity, and focused awareness. Engaging in these activities regularly has been linked to lower stress levels and enhanced general well-being.

People with IBS need to experiment with different stress-reduction strategies to see what suits them best. A customized stress-reduction strategy could incorporate therapeutic therapies, mindfulness exercises, and leisure activities that suit each person's interests.

To sum up, controlling IBS symptoms mostly depends on practicing effective stress management. The general well-being of people with IBS can be greatly improved by putting strategies like mind-body practices, cognitive-behavioral therapy, and mindfulness meditation into practice.

How Sleep Hygiene Affects IBS

It is impossible to emphasize how important getting enough sleep is to overall health, especially for those with Irritable Bowel Syndrome (IBS). Managing the symptoms of IBS requires careful consideration of sleep hygiene, which includes behaviors and routines that encourage peaceful sleep. While getting enough restorative sleep improves general well-being, sleep interruptions might make gastrointestinal problems worse.

IBS and sleep have a reciprocal relationship. IBS symptoms including pain and discomfort in the abdomen can, on the one hand, interfere with sleep cycles and make it harder to get asleep and stay asleep. Conversely, inadequate or substandard sleep can exacerbate pain sensitivity, elevate stress levels, and adversely impact digestive processes, all of which can exacerbate symptoms of IBS.

For those with IBS, it's essential to have a regular sleep schedule. The body's internal clock is regulated when you go to bed and wake up at the same time every day, which improves the quality of your sleep. It is equally crucial to create a peaceful and pleasant sleeping environment. Maintaining healthy spinal alignment entails keeping the bedroom cool, quiet, and dark in addition to investing in pillows and a comfy mattress.

For people with IBS, it's critical to limit stimulants like caffeine and nicotine in the hours before bed. These drugs may worsen gastrointestinal problems and interfere with sleep cycles. Similarly, limiting large meals close to bedtime can help reduce the likelihood of experiencing indigestion and discomfort at night.

Before going to bed, practicing relaxation techniques might be very helpful for those who have IBS. The body can be prompted to wind down and promote more restful sleep by participating in techniques like progressive muscle relaxation, mild stretching, or a relaxing bedtime ritual.

Finally, for people with IBS to properly manage their symptoms, they must prioritize good sleep hygiene. Healthy sleep practices can help people establish a sleep environment that promotes restorative sleep, which will improve their physical and mental health in general.

CHAPTER SEVEN

DIETARY STRATEGIES FOR IBS MANAGEMENT
Low-FODMAP Diet Explained:

The Low-FODMAP diet is a therapy approach that is essential to managing Irritable Bowel Syndrome (IBS). It focuses on lowering the consumption of particular fermentable carbohydrates. Fermentable oligosaccharides, disaccharides, monosaccharides, and polyols, or FODMAPs, are a class of carbohydrates that, in sensitive people, may cause gastrointestinal distress. There are three stages to the low-FODMAP diet: personalization, reintroduction, and restriction.

To ease symptoms, people remove items high in fructooligosaccharides (FODMAPS) from their diets during the restriction phase. Some fruits, vegetables, cereals, and dairy products are frequently the guilty parties. This stage is intended to be a brief intervention to pinpoint particular triggers rather than a long-term fix. To determine whether FODMAPs are troublesome, the reintroduction step entails methodically reintroducing each one at a time. Ultimately, the personalization stage enables people to modify their diet to their unique dietary sensitivity, resulting in a customized and long-lasting strategy for treating IBS.

Studies have demonstrated that the low-FODMAP diet can help with IBS symptoms; many people report notable reductions in bloating, pain in the abdomen, and general well-being. To ensure correct execution and avoid nutritional deficits, people must follow this diet plan under the supervision of a medical practitioner or a trained dietitian.

Customized Dietary Programs:

Given the distinctive characteristics of IBS and its triggers, a nutrition strategy that is tailored to each individual may not be sufficient to provide noticeable relief. Therefore, creating customized nutrition regimens is crucial to adjusting dietary approaches to each IBS patient's unique requirements. These programs consider the patient's symptom patterns and triggers in addition to their food choices and limits.

The first step in creating a customized nutrition plan for someone with IBS is usually doing a thorough evaluation of the patient's food preferences, lifestyle choices, and symptom profile. This makes it possible for medical experts to pinpoint possible triggers and create a customized strategy—often in conjunction with qualified nutritionists. The strategy can call for adjustments to overall dietary patterns, fiber types, and the consumption of particular nutrients.

Individualized nutrition programs also cover more than just meal selections. They take into account things like the timing of meals, serving amounts, and how stress affects digestion. Personalized regimens are designed to target the specific elements that contribute to each individual's IBS to offer long-lasting, sustainable treatment.

People can take an active role in their health when they are empowered to manage their symptoms through customized nutrition. It promotes a deeper comprehension of the complex relationship between food and IBS symptoms, empowering people to make decisions that improve their general well-being and standard of living.

The Brain-Gut Relationship In Eating Decisions:

The complex interaction between the brain and the gut affects the onset and intensity of IBS symptoms. The relationship between the stomach and the brain highlights the effects of stress, emotions, and mental health on digestive health, which is why nutritional approaches to controlling IBS must take this relationship into account.

IBS symptoms can be made worse by stress and emotional variables, which increases a person's risk of experiencing digestive discomfort. There is a reciprocal relationship between the gut and emotions and stress levels. It is crucial to comprehend this dynamic interaction to create dietary plans that effectively control IBS.

The gut-brain link highlights the significance of mindful eating and stress management about dietary choices. Stress-reduction methods that improve gut health and lessen symptoms of IBS include deep breathing exercises, meditation, and regular physical activity. Furthermore, adopting habits that include stress-reduction techniques can improve the efficacy of nutritional therapies.

Furthermore, the gut-brain axis draws attention to the possible influence of specific foods on stress and mood. For instance, eating foods high in probiotics may have a beneficial effect on gut flora and enhance mental health. For those with IBS, incorporating a range of nutrient-dense foods that promote both mental and digestive health becomes a crucial part of dietary recommendations.

By acknowledging and tackling the gut-brain connection in dietary decisions, people can embrace comprehensive strategies for managing IBS. By combining dietary changes with stress-reduction techniques, a complete approach that tackles the complex character of IBS is created, enhancing general health and quality of life.

CHAPTER EIGHT

DRUGS AND TREATMENTS
Options Available to Treat Irritable Bowel Syndrome (IBS)

Options that are available over-the-counter (OTC) are essential for relieving the symptoms of Irritable Bowel Syndrome (IBS). These readily available over-the-counter drugs are frequently used as first-line treatments for mild to moderate IBS symptoms. Supplemental fiber is one OTC option that is frequently used. These supplements, which come in powder, capsule, and chewable tablet formats, help relieve constipation, a common symptom of IBS and encourage regular bowel movements.

Another group of over-the-counter (OTC) treatments that address the pain and cramping in the abdomen linked to IBS is antispasmodic drugs. These drugs ease discomfort by assisting in the relaxation of the digestive tract's muscles. Furthermore, laxatives could be suggested for those with IBS who are constipation-dominant because they can assist in softening stools and making bowel motions easier.

Probiotics are becoming more and more common over-the-counter (OTC) treatments for IBS symptoms. They can be found in the form of pills, yogurt, or fermented foods. These supplements include good bacteria that support a balanced gut microbiome, which may enhance the digestion process and lessen symptoms like gas and bloating.

Even while some IBS sufferers find comfort in over-the-counter (OTC) solutions, people need to speak with healthcare providers before self-medicating. Based on the patient's unique needs and symptoms, a healthcare professional can assist in identifying the best over-the-counter solutions.

The Impact Of Prescription Drugs On Irritable Bowel Syndrome (IBS) Treatment

Prescription drugs are frequently an essential part of the treatment approach for people with more severe or resistant Irritable Bowel Syndrome (IBS) symptoms. Antispasmodics are one family of prescription drugs that are often given for IBS. These medications, which include hyoscyamine and dicyclomine, reduce cramping and pain in the abdomen by relaxing the muscles of the digestive tract.

Healthcare professionals may recommend drugs like loperamide, which reduces urgency and slows down bowel movements when diarrhea is the main symptom. On the other hand, drugs like linaclotide or lubiprostone may be suggested to encourage bowel regularity in people with IBS who are primarily constipated.

Another class of prescription drugs used to treat IBS includes selective serotonin reuptake inhibitors (SSRIs) and tricyclic antidepressants. These drugs can help control mood and alter pain signals in the gut, treating both the psychological and physical components of IBS symptoms.

People who are taking prescription drugs for IBS must carefully adhere to the directions provided by their healthcare provider and promptly report any side effects or concerns. Consultations with medical professionals regularly enable treatment plans to be modified in response to patient reactions.

Research And New Therapies In The Treatment Of Irritable Bowel Syndrome (IBS)

The therapy of Irritable Bowel Syndrome (IBS) is a constantly changing field, with novel medications and continual research providing hope for those with this chronic gastrointestinal illness. Investigating gut-directed hypnotherapy is one exciting field of study. Through the use of suggestion, this psychological intervention seeks to address the mind-gut link, lessen symptoms of IBS, and possibly even ease pain and discomfort in the abdomen.

In addition, research on IBS is focusing on the topic of microbiome modulation. Researchers are currently examining the potential benefits of probiotics, prebiotics, and fecal microbiota transplantation

(FMT) on the balance of gut bacteria and, consequently, on the improvement of IBS symptoms. Specifically, FMT transfers fecal matter from a donor who is in good health to the recipient to improve the gut microbial ecology.

Transcutaneous electrical nerve stimulation (TENS) is one neuromodulation approach that is being investigated as a possible treatment for IBS. TENS works by applying low-voltage electrical currents to particular body parts to control nerve activity and lessen IBS-related pain signals.

Although these new treatments appear promising, it's crucial to remember that more studies are required to determine their long-term efficacy and safety. As knowledge of IBS expands, people may expect more specialized and individualized approaches to treating this complicated illness, which will give hope to those who are struggling with its difficult symptoms.

CHAPITRE NINE

DIFFERENT AND SUPPLEMENTARY METHODS
The Use of Probiotics and Professional Advice in the Management of Irritable Bowel Syndrome (IBS)

Probiotics have become a viable substitute strategy for treating Irritable Bowel Syndrome (IBS). These live microbes, often known as "good bacteria," are recognized to offer several health advantages, especially when it comes to preserving the equilibrium of the gut microbiota. An imbalance in the gut microbiota causes symptoms like bloating, irregular bowel habits, and abdominal pain in people with IBS. Probiotics work by bringing good bacteria back into the digestive system to try and restore this equilibrium.

Studies indicate that some probiotic strains, such as Lactobacillus and Bifidobacterium, may reduce symptoms of irritable bowel syndrome by enhancing the function of the intestinal barrier and reducing inflammation. These microbes work by changing the gut microbiota's makeup and interacting with the immune system. Probiotics may also lessen discomfort in the abdomen and help control bowel motions in IBS sufferers.

It's critical to have professional advice before adding probiotics to an IBS treatment plan. Medical practitioners can offer tailored advice based on each patient's unique requirements and symptoms. An in-depth knowledge of the patient's health situation and any potential drug interactions is necessary to choose the best probiotic strain, dosage, and length of supplementation.

It is noteworthy that although probiotics have potential in the management of IBS symptoms, individual differences may exist in their efficaciousness. While some people could feel a great sense of relief, others might not feel the same way. Patients and healthcare professionals must work together continuously as this field of study develops to track results and make necessary corrections.

Using Traditional Medicine and Herbal Supplements to Treat Irritable Bowel Syndrome (IBS) Under Expert Guidance

For ages, herbal supplements and traditional medicine have been essential parts of healthcare systems across the globe. These days, they are becoming more and more recognized as viable options for treating Irritable Bowel Syndrome (IBS). Using botanicals, herbs, and traditional treatments for IBS seeks to improve overall digestive health and treat symptoms naturally.

Some botanicals, including turmeric, ginger, and peppermint oil, have shown promise in reducing the symptoms of IBS. For instance, peppermint oil is well-known for its antispasmodic qualities, which can aid in gastrointestinal tract muscle relaxation and lessen bloating and pain in the abdomen. The anti-inflammatory properties of ginger may help alleviate symptoms, and studies have been done on the potential of the curcumin component in turmeric to modify inflammatory pathways in the stomach.

Because the effectiveness and interactions of various natural therapies might vary, seeking expert counsel is essential when considering herbal supplements for IBS. Healthcare providers with expertise in integrative medicine can guide patients through a wide range of herbal alternatives, considering things like a patient's unique sensitivity profile, degree of symptoms, and possible drug interactions.

Ayurveda and Traditional Chinese Medicine (TCM) are two examples of traditional medical systems that provide comprehensive methods for treating the underlying imbalances that cause IBS. When customizing therapies, practitioners in these professions frequently take into account a patient's unique constitution, lifestyle, and dietary preferences. Working together with specialists in conventional medicine can offer people with IBS a thorough and customized approach to controlling their illness.

Using Acupuncture and Mind-Body Techniques Under Professional Guidance to Manage Irritable Bowel Syndrome (IBS)

More people are becoming aware of acupuncture and mind-body techniques as complementary therapies for Irritable Bowel Syndrome (IBS). These methods, which have their roots in conventional medical systems, emphasize the connection between the body and mind to reestablish equilibrium and reduce symptoms.

A crucial part of Traditional Chinese Medicine (TCM) is acupuncture, which stimulates qi flow by inserting tiny needles into predetermined body sites. According to studies, acupuncture may help people with IBS feel better by regulating gastrointestinal function, lowering inflammation, and changing how they perceive pain. To guarantee that the right acupuncture points are chosen and that treatment frequency is customized to each patient's needs, professional advice from qualified acupuncturists is crucial.

Mindfulness meditation, yoga, and cognitive-behavioral therapy (CBT) are examples of mind-body activities that emphasize the relationship between mental and physical health. These techniques seek to induce relaxation and lessen stress, which is known to be a trigger for IBS symptoms. It is essential to seek expert assistance when integrating mind-body techniques into an IBS management plan since they may offer tailored tactics and support for cultivating mindfulness.

People with IBS can investigate holistic therapies that address both the physiological and psychological elements of their problem by working with specialists in acupuncture and mind-body practices. When incorporated into a thorough treatment plan, these therapies can potentially improve the quality of life and general well-being of those with IBS.

CHAPTER TEN

EMOTIONAL HEALTH AND COPING MECHANISMS
Handling the Psychological Effects of IBS

Living with Irritable Bowel Syndrome (IBS) has a substantial emotional cost in addition to its physical difficulties. The erratic nature of symptoms associated with IBS, including bloating, irregular bowel movements, and stomach pain, can exacerbate anxiety and stress. Managing the psychological effects of IBS requires a multimodal strategy that takes into account an individual's physical symptoms as well as their mental health.

A critical component of emotional coping is realizing and comprehending how stress and IBS symptoms interact. Emotional distress can be significantly reduced with the help of stress management practices like progressive muscle relaxation, mindfulness, and deep breathing exercises. Additionally, getting help from mental health specialists like psychologists or counselors can give people coping mechanisms customized to their unique emotional struggles.

Moreover, alterations in lifestyle are crucial for the mental welfare of individuals suffering from IBS. Eating a healthy, balanced diet, exercising frequently, and getting enough sleep can all have a favorable effect on one's physical and mental well-being. An emotionally stable condition can be achieved by establishing a schedule that includes self-care activities like taking up a hobby, going for walks in the park, or practicing relaxation techniques.

Another essential component of managing the emotional effects of IBS is learning how to communicate effectively. Open communication about worries and emotions with loved ones, friends, and medical professionals creates a supportive atmosphere and improves comprehension of the difficulties encountered. Additionally, assertiveness training can enable people to effectively express their requirements, guaranteeing that their emotional health comes first.

In summary, managing the emotional effects of IBS calls for a comprehensive strategy that takes stress reduction, lifestyle adjustments, and efficient communication into account. Through the implementation of these tactics in their daily lives, people with IBS can develop emotional resilience and enhance their general quality of life.

Peer Links and Support Groups

Managing the difficulties caused by Irritable Bowel Syndrome (IBS) can be a solitary journey; yet, seeking comfort in support groups and forming relationships with peers can significantly impact one's experience. Individuals with IBS can discuss their experiences, trade coping mechanisms, and offer mutual understanding in a nonjudgmental setting by joining support groups.

Joining a support group helps people feel less alone when dealing with chronic illnesses by providing a sense of community. Knowing they are not alone in their battles with IBS might give them strength. Within the group, sharing personal experiences promotes empathy and camaraderie, forming a supporting network that is essential to mental health.

Within these groups, peer relationships add to a common body of information regarding the management of IBS symptoms. Individuals frequently share helpful advice on dietary changes, stress management methods, and lifestyle alterations. For those looking to enhance their quality of life while managing IBS, this body of knowledge—which is derived from actual experiences—can be quite helpful.

In addition, support groups provide forums for learning, where participants can learn about the most recent studies, available treatments, and coping mechanisms. By exchanging knowledge among members of the group, people are better equipped to make educated healthcare decisions and effectively manage their IBS.

In conclusion, peer relationships and support groups provide a lifeline for people struggling with IBS. By offering emotional support, a forum for exchanging experiences, and useful information, these communities help people manage the difficulties presented by IBS in a more knowledgeable and resilient manner.

Developing Resilience and Keeping an Upbeat Attitude

Developing resilience and keeping an optimistic outlook are crucial elements of managing Irritable Bowel Syndrome (IBS) well. IBS symptoms can be emotionally draining because they are chronic, therefore people must develop resilience so they can deal with the highs and lows of their health journey.

Being resilient is overcoming obstacles and adjusting to hardship. For those who have IBS, this entails creating coping strategies that enable them to face the unknowns of their illness head-on with courage and resolve. Due to their ability to foster a present-focused mentality and lessen the influence of negative thoughts and emotions, mindfulness exercises like yoga and meditation can be effective techniques for developing resilience.

Resilience and maintaining a positive outlook are strongly related. It entails developing optimism in the face of long-term health difficulties. To encourage a more optimistic view and alter negative thought patterns, cognitive-behavioral approaches might be especially useful. Furthermore, cultivating a positive outlook and finding delight in the little things in life, along with practicing appreciation, support emotional well-being.

Acknowledging and accepting the restrictions imposed by IBS while concentrating on factors under one's control is a critical component of developing resilience. This entails setting reasonable objectives, acknowledging minor victories, and appreciating the advancements gained in symptom management. People can improve their capacity to manage the psychological and physical difficulties associated with IBS by embracing an empowered and proactive mentality.

To sum up, developing resilience and keeping an optimistic outlook are essential elements of an all-encompassing strategy for controlling IBS. By engaging in mindfulness exercises, cognitive-behavioral therapy, and a growth-oriented approach, people can develop the emotional resilience required to flourish despite the difficulties presented by IBS.

CHAPTER ELEVEN

PROSPECTIVE PATTERNS AND DEVELOPMENTS IN IBS STUDIES
State of IBS Research Right Now:

The topic of Irritable Bowel Syndrome (IBS) research has been lively and multifaceted as of my previous knowledge update in January 2022, marked by continued efforts to decipher the intricate mechanisms behind this gastrointestinal condition.

Numerous topics have been explored by researchers, including the composition of the microbiome, the gut-brain axis, and the function of immune responses in IBS. IBS has come to be recognized as a functional gastrointestinal condition, recognizing the complex interaction between physiological and psychological components.

Technological developments have made it possible to use increasingly complex diagnostic tools, like molecular diagnostics and improved imaging, which have given researchers a better understanding of the pathophysiology of IBS.

One area of focus has been the discovery of certain biomarkers linked to various IBS subtypes, which has made it possible to develop more specialized and individualized treatment plans. Genetic research has also helped to identify the genetic predispositions that may make an individual more susceptible to IBS.

Even with advancements, IBS is still difficult to identify a single causative factor for because of its variability and range of clinical manifestations. The dearth of medicines that work for everyone highlights the need for a more sophisticated comprehension of unique patient profiles.

Positive Advancements and Clinical Research:

Novel therapy methods and an increase in clinical studies investigating creative ways to control IBS symptoms are two encouraging recent developments. The regulation of the gut microbiota is one prominent topic of focus.

To improve microbial balance and reduce symptoms, research has been done on probiotics, prebiotics, and fecal microbiota transplantation (FMT). Positive early results from a few trials have raised hopes for the potential of medicines targeted to the microbiota.

In addition, neuro-modulation methods such as brain stimulation and biofeedback have drawn interest as possible treatments for the dysregulation of the gut-brain axis associated with IBS. With any luck, symptoms can be managed. These methods work by altering neuronal signals and improving brain-to-gastrointestinal tract connection.

Drugs that target particular receptors and neurotransmitters linked to IBS are the focus of ongoing clinical trials investigating pharmacological treatments. The creation of drugs that target the psychological and gastrointestinal aspects of IBS is a reflection of our growing comprehension of its complex nature.

The Way Ahead: Hope for Those with IBS:

The future of care for those with IBS is marked by a growing trend toward individualized and comprehensive approaches. Integrative methods, which take into account the connection between mental and physical health, are becoming more and more popular. It is acknowledged that dietary changes, stress reduction techniques, and lifestyle adjustments are crucial elements of holistic IBS care.

Empowerment and education of patients are crucial in this changing environment. As more information regarding the specific character of IBS becomes available, individuals will be able to actively engage in the treatment process and make decisions based on their symptom profiles and preferences.

Furthermore, the advent of digital health tools and telemedicine has made it easier to monitor and help patients remotely, improving access to professional advice. This makes it possible to provide more ongoing, individualized care that is tailored to the various needs of people with IBS.

In summary:

To sum up, there is hope for IBS research in the future thanks to the development of focused therapies and a better knowledge of its intricate etiology. To overcome IBS, a multidisciplinary strategy that incorporates knowledge from psychology, neurology, gastrointestinal, and other pertinent disciplines must be adopted. IBS patients now have more optimism thanks to continuing clinical trials, technology advancements, and a greater emphasis on individualized care. As we commemorate the advancements of the past year, patients, healthcare providers, and researchers must work together to shape a future in which the burden of IBS is much reduced, if not completely abolished.

www.ingramcontent.com/pod-product-compliance
Lightning Source LLC
Chambersburg PA
CBHW050742260726
48661CB00001B/363